Natural Cleaners for Your Home

Homemade Recipes On A Budget

Table of Contents

Introduction

There you are, standing in another aisle, and trying to find a cleaner you feel comfortable using around your home. You love it when your house is clean and sanitized, and nothing makes you happier than seeing the shine in your bathroom, on your tile, and over your appliances.

But, as you read over the ingredient lists, you see warning after warning to keep the cleaners away from your kids and your pets. Though you know you can keep them out of reach, you wonder if it is truly worth exposing your loved ones to such chemicals.

Not only that, but these cleaners are expensive, and you spend more money trying to keep the bathroom clean than you spend on the bathroom itself.

If only there was a way for you to enjoy a clean and sanitized house without breaking the bank. If only there was a way for you to know what is in the cleaners, and know without a doubt that they aren't going to harm your kids or your pets.

If only there was a way for you to make the cleaners yourself.

Now, there is.

With this book, you are going to learn the recipes you need to clean around your home without worry. You are about to discover the secret to the perfectly clean house, without having to expose yourself or any of your loved ones to harmful chemicals.

The recipes in this book are perfect for anyone who wants to save money, do the environment a favor, and have peace of mind that they are not exposing themselves or their loved ones to any harmful chemicals.

This book is full of these recipes, and will provide you with the perfect cleaners to cleanse your bathroom, kitchen, and virtually anywhere else in your home – and even you!

You will fall in love with each and every one of these recipes, and experience a clean like you never have before.

So, are you ready to clean things the right way?

Good.

Let's get started.

Chapter 1 – Bathroom Cleaners

The bathroom is perhaps the germiest place in the entire house, and it needs to be cleaned thoroughly. But, so many bathroom cleaners are filled with chemicals and harmful additives that you don't want around you, your pets, or your kids.

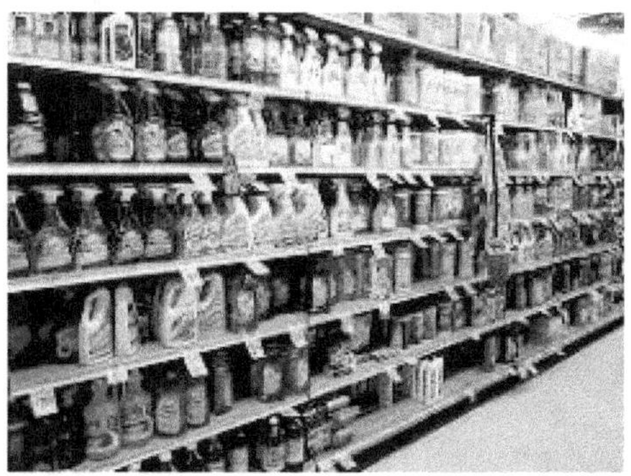

With these cleaners, you can rest assured that you are only harming the germs, and nothing else. Mix them all and use them all over your bathroom, and enjoy cleaning in a whole new way.

Sparkle and Shine Shower Cleaner
You will need:

¾ cup baking soda

4 tablespoons salt

½ cup vinegar

½ cup warm water

1/3 cup lemon juice

15 drops lemon essential oil

Directions:

Use a large bowl, as the combination of vinegar and baking soda will cause a reaction. After you have mixed all the ingredients well, use a funnel to pour them into a bottle for use.

To use:

This mix is too thick to spray out of a bottle, so pour it directly onto your towel or cleaning cloth and scrub your shower that way.

Tub Scrub

What you will need:

1 bottle hydrogen peroxide

Iodized sea salt

Directions:

Pour the bottle of hydrogen peroxide into a large dish, then stir in the salt. Continue to add the salt until you have a paste.

To use:

Use the entire mix in your bathtub at a time, scrubbing well. Allow the solution to sit in the tub for half an hour, then rinse with hot water.

Bathroom Shiner
What you will need:

1 cup baking soda

½ cup castile soap

2 tablespoons warm water

10 drops peppermint essential oil

Directions:

Use a large bowl to combine the ingredients, and use the entire batch when you clean your bathroom.

Begin with combining the baking soda and castile soap, then stir in the peppermint oil. Slowly add the warm water, until you reach a paste like consistency.

To use:

Pour the mix directly onto your washcloth, or directly onto the surface you wish to clean. Use a sponge or a scrubber to scrub well, then allow to sit for a few minutes before wiping off.

Perfectly Shined Grout Scrub
What you will need:

What you will need:

1 bottle hydrogen peroxide

1 carton baking soda (use the large box so you have enough to create a paste)

Directions:

Pour the bottle of hydrogen peroxide into a large dish, then stir in the baking soda. Continue to add the baking soda until you have a paste.

To use:

Apply generously to the grout in your bathroom, and allow to sit for a few minutes. Use a sponge or cleaning towel to scrub vigorously, then use another cleaning towel to wipe off the residue.

Germ Be Gone Toilet Cleaner

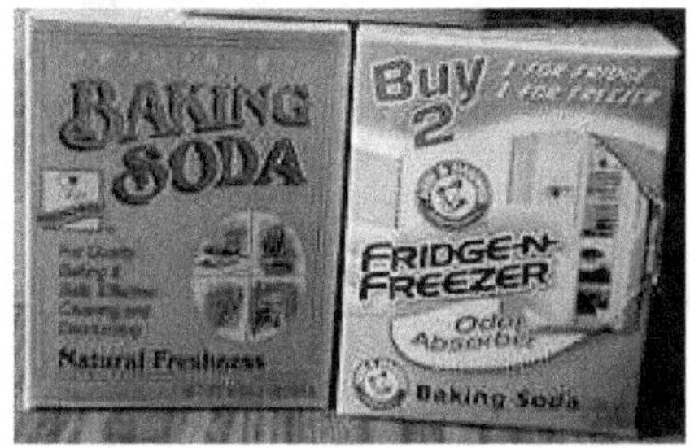

What you will need:

1 cup baking soda

½ cup vinegar

10 drops orange oil

10 drops lemon oil

10 drops lemongrass oil

Directions:

Pour all ingredients directly into your toilet bowl.

To use:

Use your toilet brush to vigorously scrub your toil bowl, with all the ingredients inside. Allow to sit in the toilet for 10 to 20 minutes, then flush. Repeat as needed.

Anti-bacterial Bathroom Cleanse
What you will need:

½ cup vodka

1 cup vinegar

½ cup lemon juice

10 drops orange essential oil

10 drops lemon essential oil

10 drops lavender essential oil

1 cup water

Directions:

Mix all ingredients well, then transfer into a spray bottle.

To use:

Shake well before each use, and spray generously on any surface in the bathroom you like. Use your sponge or cleaning cloth to scrub the surface, then dry thoroughly.

Repeat as needed.

Chapter 2 – Glass and Surface Cleaners

There are few things more annoying than streaky glass or a mirror you can't see into. These blends are going to solve this problem for you, giving you the clarity you yearn for without exposing anyone to anything harmful.

Try them all and decide which is your favorite, and never turn back to the store chemicals again.

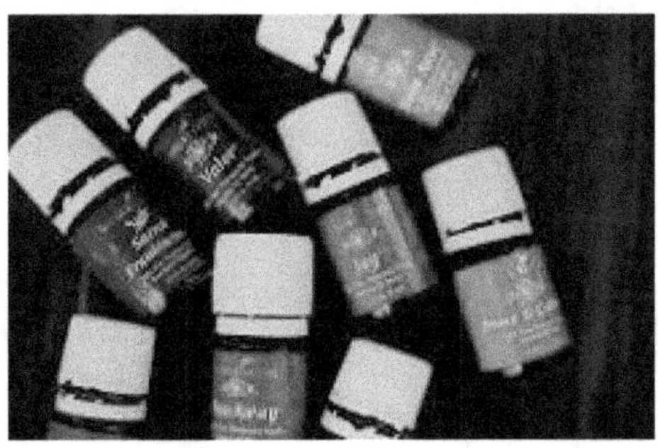

Minty Mirrors
What you will need:

10 drops peppermint oil

10 drops spearmint oil

10 drops eucalyptus oil

1 cup vinegar

Warm water

Directions:

Combine all ingredients and transfer to a spray bottle. Fill the remaining portion of the bottle with water, and shake well before each use.

To use:

Spray generously over your mirror or windows, then wipe clean with a cloth. Repeat as often as needed.

Streak Free Clean and Shine
What you will need:

20 drops orange oil

10 drops blood orange oil

10 drops lemon oil

1 cup vinegar

Warm water

Directions:

Combine all ingredients and transfer to a spray bottle. Fill the remaining portion of the bottle with water, and shake well before each use.

To use:

Spray generously over your mirror or windows, then wipe clean with a cloth. Repeat as often as needed.

Love Yourself Mirror Cleaner
What you will need:

10 drops tea tree oil

10 drops clary sage oil

1 cup vinegar

Warm water

Directions:

Combine all ingredients and transfer to a spray bottle. Fill the remaining portion of the bottle with water, and shake well before each use.

To use:

Spray generously over your mirror or windows, then wipe clean with a cloth. Repeat as often as needed.

Clear Vision Glass Cleaner

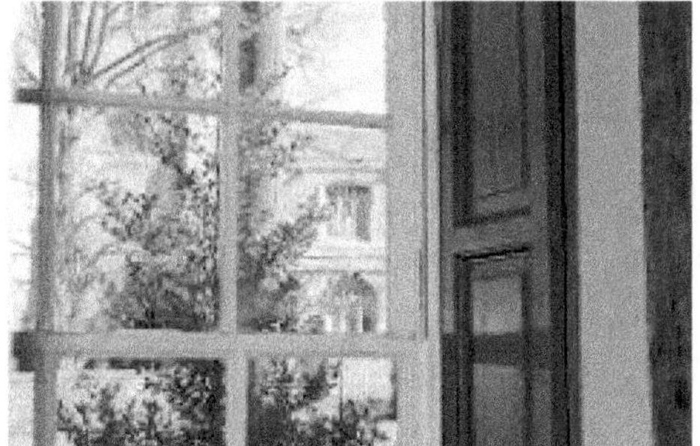

What you will need:

10 drops frankincense oil

10 drops myrrh oil

10 drops goldenseal oil

1 cup vinegar

Warm water

Directions:

Combine all ingredients and transfer to a spray bottle. Fill the remaining portion of the bottle with water, and shake well before each use.

To use:

Spray generously over your mirror or windows, then wipe clean with a cloth. Repeat as often as needed.

Safe and Effective Surface Cleaner
What you will need:

10 drops lavender oil

10 drops orange oil

10 drops eucalyptus oil

1 cup vinegar

Warm water

Directions:

Combine all ingredients and transfer to a spray bottle. Fill the remaining portion of the bottle with water, and shake well before each use.

To use:

Spray generously over your mirror or windows, then wipe clean with a cloth. Repeat as often as needed.

Everything's Clean Scented Cleaner
What you will need:

10 drops geranium oil

10 drops tea tree oil

10 drops clary sage oil

1 cup vinegar

Warm water

Directions:

Combine all ingredients and transfer to a spray bottle. Fill the remaining portion of the bottle with water, and shake well before each use.

To use:

Spray generously over your mirror or windows, then wipe clean with a cloth. Repeat as often as needed.

Clear Mirror
What you will need:

10 drops sandalwood oil

10 drops tea tree oil

10 drops cinnamon oil

1 cup vinegar

Warm water

Directions:

Combine all ingredients and transfer to a spray bottle. Fill the remaining portion of the bottle with water, and shake well before each use.

To use:

Spray generously over your mirror or windows, then wipe clean with a cloth. Repeat as often as needed.

I Can See Clearly Window Spray
What you will need:

10 drops eucalyptus oil

10 drops lemongrass oil

10 drops blood orange oil

1 cup vinegar

Warm water

Directions:

Combine all ingredients and transfer to a spray bottle. Fill the remaining portion of the bottle with water, and shake well before each use.

To use:

Spray generously over your mirror or windows, then wipe clean with a cloth. Repeat as often as needed.

Where's the Window? Spray
What you will need:

10 drops wintergreen oil

10 drops blood orange oil

10 drops clary sage oil

1 cup vinegar

Warm water

Directions:

Combine all ingredients and transfer to a spray bottle. Fill the remaining portion of the bottle with water, and shake well before each use.

To use:

Spray generously over your mirror or windows, then wipe clean with a cloth. Repeat as often as needed.

Streakless Spray

What you will need:

10 drops chamomile oil

10 drops tea tree oil

10 drops peppermint oil

1 cup vinegar

Warm water

Directions:

Combine all ingredients and transfer to a spray bottle. Fill the remaining portion of the bottle with water, and shake well before each use.

To use:

Spray generously over your mirror or windows, then wipe clean with a cloth. Repeat as often as needed.

Chapter 3 – Kitchen Cleaners

It's incredibly important that your kitchen stays clean. Not only do you cook in there, but you often eat there, too. The kitchen, unfortunately, can be the site of many different kinds of germs, and must be sanitized, too.

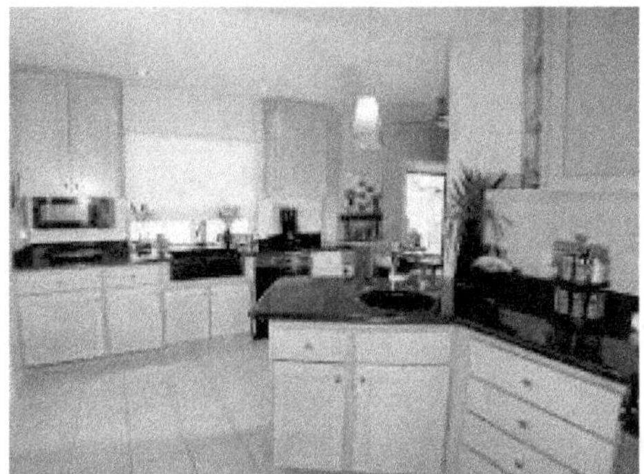

With these blends, you don't have to worry about harmful chemicals being near your food. Mix every recipe and try them for yourself. You are sure to fall in love with the results, every time.

Appliance Shiner
What you will need:

10 drops geranium oil

10 drops tea tree oil

10 drops cinnamon oil

1 cup vinegar

1 cup vodka

Warm water

2 tablespoons dish soap

Directions:

Combine all ingredients and transfer to a cleaning spray bottle. Fill the remaining space in the bottle with water, and remember to shake well before using.

To use:

Spray generously over any surface you need cleaned, then use your sponge or cleaning cloth to scrub vigorously. Repeat as often as needed.

Perfectionist Floor Cleaner

What you will need:

10 drops vanilla oil

10 drops peppermint oil

10 drops orange oil

1 cup vinegar

1 cup vodka

Warm water

2 tablespoons dish soap

Directions:

Combine all ingredients and transfer to a cleaning spray bottle. Fill the remaining space in the bottle with water, and remember to shake well before using.

To use:

Spray generously over any surface you need cleaned, then use your sponge or cleaning cloth to scrub vigorously. Repeat as often as needed.

Top of the Line All Purpose Cleaner
What you will need:

10 drops lemon oil

10 drops wheatgrass oil

10 drops eucalyptus oil

1 cup vinegar

1 cup vodka

Warm water

2 tablespoons dish soap

Directions:

Combine all ingredients and transfer to a cleaning spray bottle. Fill the remaining space in the bottle with water, and remember to shake well before using.

To use:

Spray generously over any surface you need cleaned, then use your sponge or cleaning cloth to scrub vigorously. Repeat as often as needed.

Rainy Day Scrub
What you will need:

10 drops bergamot oil

10 drops basil oil

10 drops tea tree oil

1 cup vinegar

1 cup vodka

Warm water

2 tablespoons dish soap

Directions:

Combine all ingredients and transfer to a cleaning spray bottle. Fill the remaining space in the bottle with water, and remember to shake well before using.

To use:

Spray generously over any surface you need cleaned, then use your sponge or cleaning cloth to scrub vigorously. Repeat as often as needed.

Spotless Kitchen Cleaner

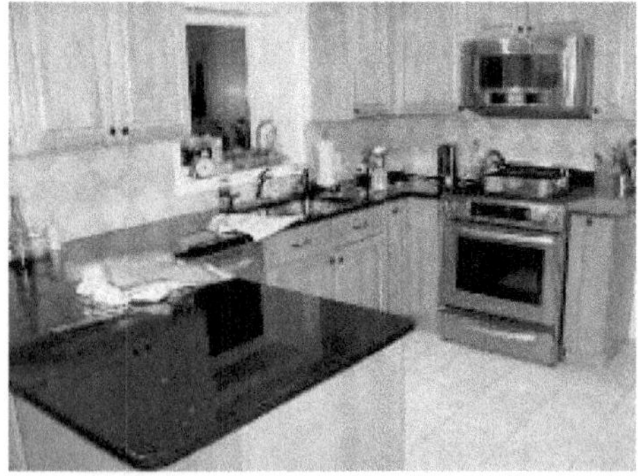

What you will need:

10 drops lemon oil

10 drops peppermint oil

10 drops lavender oil

10 drops cinnamon oil

1 cup vinegar

1 cup vodka

Warm water

2 tablespoons dish soap

Directions:

Combine all ingredients and transfer to a cleaning spray bottle. Fill the remaining space in the bottle with water, and remember to shake well before using.

To use:

Spray generously over any surface you need cleaned, then use your sponge or cleaning cloth to scrub vigorously. Repeat as often as needed.

Clean and Clear Cleaner

What you will need:

10 drops clary sage oil

10 drops orange oil

10 drops lemon oil

10 drops lemongrass oil

1 cup vinegar

1 cup vodka

Warm water

2 tablespoons dish soap

Directions:

Combine all ingredients and transfer to a cleaning spray bottle. Fill the remaining space in the bottle with water, and remember to shake well before using.

To use:

Spray generously over any surface you need cleaned, then use your sponge or cleaning cloth to scrub vigorously. Repeat as often as needed.

Food Grade Safety Cleaner
What you will need:

20 drops grapefruit oil

10 drops lemon oil

10 drops orange oil

10 drops blood orange oil

1 cup vinegar

1 cup vodka

Warm water

2 tablespoons dish soap

Directions:

Combine all ingredients and transfer to a cleaning spray bottle. Fill the remaining space in the bottle with water, and remember to shake well before using.

To use:

Spray generously over any surface you need cleaned, then use your sponge or cleaning cloth to scrub vigorously. Repeat as often as needed.

Clean Kitchen

What you will need:

10 drops peppermint oil

10 drops wintergreen oil

10 drops spearmint oil

1 cup vinegar

1 cup vodka

Warm water

2 tablespoons dish soap

Directions:

Combine all ingredients and transfer to a cleaning spray bottle. Fill the remaining space in the bottle with water, and remember to shake well before using.

To use:

Spray generously over any surface you need cleaned, then use your sponge or cleaning cloth to scrub vigorously. Repeat as often as needed.

Happy Housewife Cleaner

What you will need:

10 drops sandalwood oil

10 drops rosewood oil

10 drops cedar oil

1 cup vinegar

1 cup vodka

Warm water

2 tablespoons dish soap

Directions:

Combine all ingredients and transfer to a cleaning spray bottle. Fill the remaining space in the bottle with water, and remember to shake well before using.

To use:

Spray generously over any surface you need cleaned, then use your sponge or cleaning cloth to scrub vigorously. Repeat as often as needed.

Company's Coming Cleaner

What you will need:

10 drops cinnamon oil

10 drops geranium oil

10 drops lavender oil

10 drops orange oil

1 cup vinegar

1 cup vodka

Warm water

2 tablespoons dish soap

Directions:

Combine all ingredients and transfer to a cleaning spray bottle. Fill the remaining space in the bottle with water, and remember to shake well before using.

To use:

Spray generously over any surface you need cleaned, then use your sponge or cleaning cloth to scrub vigorously. Repeat as often as needed.

Chapter 4 – All Purpose Cleaning

There are times when it doesn't matter what you need to clean, you just need to clean. That's where these cleaners come in. Not only will you be able to kick the grime, but you're going to sanitize and rid your home of germs, too.

Without the harmful chemicals, it's okay for you to be generous with these blends, and clean up that mess.

Clean it Up

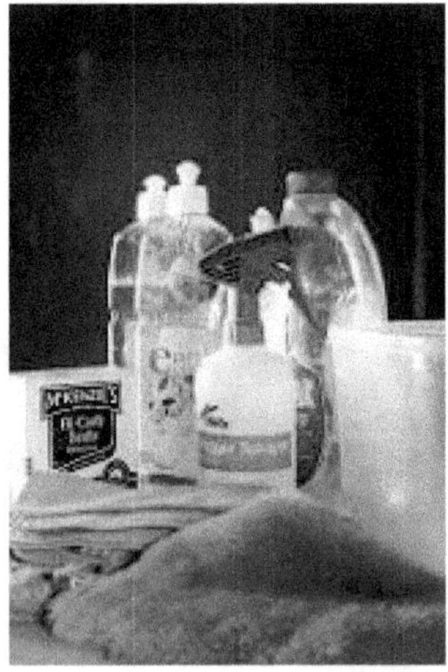

What you will need:

10 drops tea tree oil

10 drops lavender oil

10 drops lemon oil

1 cup baking soda

½ cup vodka

¼ cup vinegar

Directions:

Mix all ingredients in a large bowl and transfer to a bottle. The mixture will be too thick to spray out of the bottle, so when you are ready to use, pour directly onto the surface or onto a cleaning cloth then the surface.

To use:

Apply to any surface you need cleaned, and scrub well. Dampen another cloth and wipe any remaining residue from the surface.

Sparkling Floors and Countertops

What you will need:

10 drops clary sage oil

10 drops orange oil

10 drops blood orange oil

1 cup baking soda

½ cup vodka

¼ cup vinegar

Directions:

Mix all ingredients in a large bowl and transfer to a bottle. The mixture will be too thick to spray out of the bottle, so when you are ready to use, pour directly onto the surface or onto a cleaning cloth then the surface.

To use:

Apply to any surface you need cleaned, and scrub well. Dampen another cloth and wipe any remaining residue from the surface.

When it's Dirty

What you will need:

10 drops geranium oil

10 drops eucalyptus oil

10 drops lemon oil

1 cup baking soda

½ cup vodka

¼ cup vinegar

Directions:

Mix all ingredients in a large bowl and transfer to a bottle. The mixture will be too thick to spray out of the bottle, so when you are ready to use, pour directly onto the surface or onto a cleaning cloth then the surface.

To use:

Apply to any surface you need cleaned, and scrub well. Dampen another cloth and wipe any remaining residue from the surface.

What You've Been Waiting For

What you will need:

10 drops chamomile oil

10 drops cedar oil

10 drops sandalwood oil

1 cup baking soda

½ cup vodka

¼ cup vinegar

Directions:

Mix all ingredients in a large bowl and transfer to a bottle. The mixture will be too thick to spray out of the bottle, so when you are ready to use, pour directly onto the surface or onto a cleaning cloth then the surface.

To use:

Apply to any surface you need cleaned, and scrub well. Dampen another cloth and wipe any remaining residuc from the surface.

Clap for Clean

What you will need:

10 drops tea tree oil

10 drops basil oil

10 drops fir needle oil

1 cup baking soda

½ cup vodka

¼ cup vinegar

Directions:

Mix all ingredients in a large bowl and transfer to a bottle. The mixture will be too thick to spray out of the bottle, so when you are ready to use, pour directly onto the surface or onto a cleaning cloth then the surface.

To use:

Apply to any surface you need cleaned, and scrub well. Dampen another cloth and wipe any remaining residue from the surface.

Clean Machine

What you will need:

10 drops tea tree oil

10 drops orange oil

10 drops myrrh oil

1 cup baking soda

½ cup vodka

¼ cup vinegar

Directions:

Mix all ingredients in a large bowl and transfer to a bottle. The mixture will be too thick to spray out of the bottle, so when you are ready to use, pour directly onto the surface or onto a cleaning cloth then the surface.

To use:

Apply to any surface you need cleaned, and scrub well. Dampen another cloth and wipe any remaining residue from the surface.

Grime Be Gone

What you will need:

10 drops vetiver oil

10 drops juniper berry oil

10 drops rose oil

1 cup baking soda

½ cup vodka

¼ cup vinegar

Directions:

Mix all ingredients in a large bowl and transfer to a bottle. The mixture will be too thick to spray out of the bottle, so when you are ready to use, pour directly onto the surface or onto a cleaning cloth then the surface.

To use:

Apply to any surface you need cleaned, and scrub well. Dampen another cloth and wipe any remaining residue from the surface.

Pet Safe Cleaner
What you will need:

10 drops blood orange oil

10 drops ylang ylang oil

10 drops cedar oil

1 cup baking soda

½ cup vodka

¼ cup vinegar

Directions:

Mix all ingredients in a large bowl and transfer to a bottle. The mixture will be too thick to spray out of the bottle, so when you are ready to use, pour directly onto the surface or onto a cleaning cloth then the surface.

To use:

Apply to any surface you need cleaned, and scrub well. Dampen another cloth and wipe any remaining residue from the surface.

Fresh Air
What you will need:

10 drops tea tree oil

10 drops clary sage oil

10 drops eucalyptus oil

10 drops cinnamon oil

1 cup baking soda

½ cup vodka

¼ cup vinegar

Directions:

Mix all ingredients in a large bowl and transfer to a bottle. The mixture will be too thick to spray out of the bottle, so when you are ready to use, pour directly onto the surface or onto a cleaning cloth then the surface.

To use:

Apply to any surface you need cleaned, and scrub well. Dampen another cloth and wipe any remaining residue from the surface.

It's In the Breeze
What you will need:

10 drops grapefruit oil

10 drops lemon oil

10 drops orange oil

1 cup baking soda

½ cup vodka

¼ cup vinegar

Directions:

Mix all ingredients in a large bowl and transfer to a bottle. The mixture will be too thick to spray out of the bottle, so when you are ready to use, pour directly onto the surface or onto a cleaning cloth then the surface.

To use:

Apply to any surface you need cleaned, and scrub well. Dampen another cloth and wipe any remaining residue from the surface.

Chapter 5 – Soaps, Shampoos, and More

Cleaning isn't always about what's in the house around you. Clearly you want to be clean and healthy, too! In this final chapter, we are going to look at the mixes you can make to clean your hands, hair, and body, giving you the clear skin and shiny mane you have always wanted.

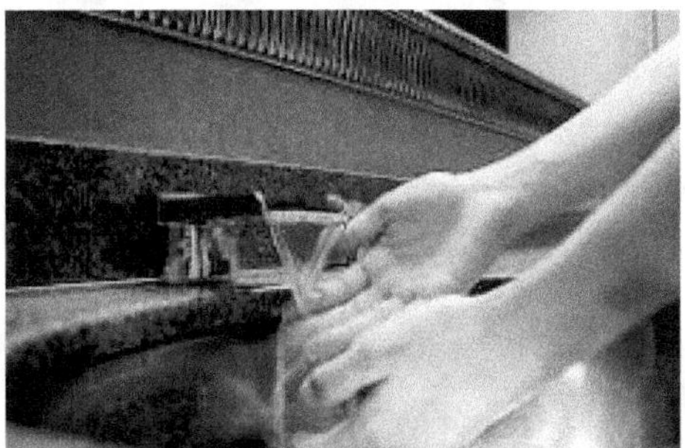

Add a little of these blends to your conventional soap, and experience a new kind of clean.

Kick the Cold Hand Soap
What you will need:

10 drops frankincense oil

10 drops orange oil

10 drops lemon oil

10 drops cinnamon oil

1 cup warm water

2 tablespoons apple cider vinegar

1 teaspoon fractionated coconut oil

Directions:

Combine all ingredients and store in a dish. Add a tablespoon to the normal soap you use to wash each time you clean.

To use:

Wash as you normally would, and make sure you rinse thoroughly with warm water.

Use every time you wash, or as often as you like.

Sleek and Shine Shampoo Blend
What you will need:

10 drops cinnamon oil

10 drops peppermint oil

10 drops orange oil

1 cup warm water

2 tablespoons apple cider vinegar

1 teaspoon fractionated coconut oil

Directions:

Combine all ingredients and store in a dish. Add a tablespoon to the normal soap you use to wash each time you clean.

To use:

Wash as you normally would, and make sure you rinse thoroughly with warm water.

Use every time you wash, or as often as you like.

Clear Skin Face Toner
What you will need:

10 drops grapefruit oil

10 drops myrrh oil

10 drops cinnamon oil

1 cup warm water

2 tablespoons apple cider vinegar

1 teaspoon fractionated coconut oil

Directions:

Combine all ingredients and store in a dish. Add a tablespoon to the normal soap you use to wash each time you clean.

To use:

Wash as you normally would, and make sure you rinse thoroughly with warm water.

Use every time you wash, or as often as you like.

Smiles Toothpaste
What you will need:

10 drops ginger oil

10 drops clove oil

10 drops cinnamon oil

½ cup baking soda

Directions:

Combine all ingredients and store in a dish. Dip your toothbrush in this paste or use with your normal toothpaste.

To use:

Brush normally, two or three times a day.

Germ Buster Soap
What you will need:

10 drops frankincense oil

10 drops myrrh oil

10 drops eucalyptus oil

1 cup warm water

2 tablespoons apple cider vinegar

1 teaspoon fractionated coconut oil

Directions:

Combine all ingredients and store in a dish. Add a tablespoon to the normal soap you use to wash each time you clean.

To use:

Wash as you normally would, and make sure you rinse thoroughly with warm water.

Use every time you wash, or as often as you like.

All Over Body Wash Blend
What you will need:

10 drops rose oil

10 drops orange oil

10 drops peppermint oil

1 cup warm water

2 tablespoons apple cider vinegar

1 teaspoon fractionated coconut oil

Directions:

Combine all ingredients and store in a dish. Add a tablespoon to the normal soap you use to wash each time you clean.

To use:

Wash as you normally would, and make sure you rinse thoroughly with warm water.

Use every time you wash, or as often as you like.

Happy Healthy Soap
What you will need:

10 drops lemon oil

10 drops cedarwood oil

10 drops cinnamon oil

1 cup warm water

2 tablespoons apple cider vinegar

1 teaspoon fractionated coconut oil

Directions:

Combine all ingredients and store in a dish. Add a tablespoon to the normal soap you use to wash each time you clean.

To use:

Wash as you normally would, and make sure you rinse thoroughly with warm water.

Use every time you wash, or as often as you like.

Give a Hand Soap

What you will need:

10 drops myrrh oil

10 drops ginger oil

10 drops geranium oil

1 cup warm water

2 tablespoons apple cider vinegar

1 teaspoon fractionated coconut oil

Directions:

Combine all ingredients and store in a dish. Add a tablespoon to the normal soap you use to wash each time you clean.

To use:

Wash as you normally would, and make sure you rinse thoroughly with warm water.

Use every time you wash, or as often as you like.

Conclusion

There you have it, everything you need to know to make your own cleansers and soaps. I hope this book was able to inspire you to take a step back from the commercial cleansers that are filled with harmful chemicals, and make a decision that is good for your family, good for your budget, and good for the environment.

When you make the decision to mix your own cleaners, you are not only doing something right for yourself, but you are also helping ease the burden of harmful chemicals on the world around you. Companies that produce those cleaners are harming the environment in a variety of ways, and the more you can step out of that, the better.

Not only are you going to be able to rest easy knowing that you aren't exposing yourself or your loved ones to these chemicals, but you are also saving money. We all know how pricy household cleaners can be, and when you step into the world of shampoos and conditioners, things are even more expensive.

Anything you can do to prevent you or your family from being exposed to these chemicals will have a wonderful impact on your health in the long run. Not only are you going to be sick less often, but you don't have to worry about the effects of these chemicals on your skin.

You don't have to worry about what would happen if your children were to get into the mix, and you don't have to worry that your pets are being exposed when they are licking their paws.

When you make your own cleaners, you are doing your whole family a wonderful service. Then, when you realize how much money you are saving, you will fall in love with them even more.

Once you try these cleaners out for yourself, you aren't ever going to want to go back to the store bought chemicals. You will discover that these clean just as well, and cost a fraction of the price.

They give you peace of mind, and they are effective – the perfect combination for anyone who is concerned with the additives in modern cleansers. Now get out there and start mixing and get to work.

Your house will be cleaner than ever, the safe way.